Paleo Diet For Beginners - The Complete Paleo Diet Guide Including 21 Delicious Paleo Recipes!

Praise For "Paleo Diet For Beginners":

Since I've read the book, I have honestly felt the best I ever can remember without doing unnecessary dieting "tricks". The eating habits it has taught me have truly been instrumental in living a healthier lifestyle... I highly recommend this book. Trust me... it's the best one around!
- Nick ★★★★★

I really enjoyed reading about why certain foods are bad for us, instead of just being told not to eat them. I loved the grocery list! Starting this lifestyle change has been challenging, and I think the list will help a lot!
- Chelsea ★★★★★

I have never been a big fan of the word "diet", because when I hear that word I automatically think of restriction and short-term gimmicks...A few of the benefits I've seen from implementing this

program (even in the few days I have been following it) has been: increased energy, less cravings for sugar & fake sweeteners, improved ability to focus on tasks, and weight loss. The day-to-day recipes are delicious and easy to follow, but the dessert recipes are an added bonus for a person such as myself who loves a treat after a long day of eating healthy. You won't find a better guide than this to jumpstart your healthier lifestyle goals for 2013.
- Brittany F. ★★★★★

-22 Pounds in two months!

I stumbled on this book after I'd already started Paleo. Taylor is right, it isn't a diet, but rather a lifestyle that is easily maintained and healthy at the same time. This book is short and to the point. The physiology of the impact certain foods have on the human body are explained without the scientific boring detail. Taylor provides an easy to follow daily routine to get you started and includes some menus and shopping lists to take the sting out of trying this revolutionary approach to a healthy lifestyle.

It is working for me and I'm not about to stop. I'm looking forward to summer when I can finally take off my shirt without feeling subconscious!
- PDX ★★★★★

Disclaimer

The techniques, strategies, and all suggestions within this book and text are intended for your educational purposes only. The author and publisher are in no way rendering medical advice of any kind, nor is this book intended to replace medical advice, nor to diagnose, prescribe or treat any disease, condition, illness or injury. The author and publisher claim no responsibility to any person or entity for any liability, loss, or damage caused, or alleged to be caused, directly or indirectly as a result of use, application or interpretation of the material in this text.

FREE Paleo Breakfast Recipe Book!

For a limited time I am giving away my Best Selling Paleo Breakfast Recipe Book for FREE! Yes, that's right... head to **FreeBookGift.com** now!

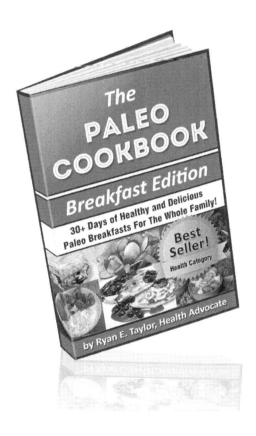

More Best Sellers That Compliment The Paleo Diet:

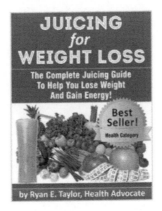

GO Here--> **FCRW.org/juicing**

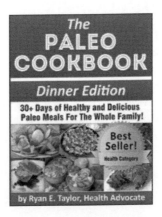

GO Here--> **FCRW.org/dinner**

Table of Contents

Introduction

The Paleo diet is a diet unlike any other diet out there - because the Paleo Diet IS NOT a diet!! Yes, you heard that right. I actually hate the concept of a diet, and I have a sneaking suspicion that you do as well. The Paleo Diet is a LIFESTYLE and once you see the light - or in this case, feel the light, you might just give up all of those bad foods for good. I'll show you the way and hold your hand through this journey, but first, a little story on how I got into this crazy world of Paleo...

My Story

My story isn't overly complicated. I grew up eating decently healthy, but I also drank soda, ate sugary sweets, consumed processed foods, and even chowed down on fast food (yikes!). One day I was given a CD of a talk on eating a clean, pure diet. I had no idea this CD would send me on the ultimate health journey over the next few years. The speaker explained things like "eating organic" and "eating living foods." It seemed like foreign talk at the time but it started to make a lot sense as I continued to listen.

At the end of the CD, the speaker encouraged the audience to try eating clean for 30 days and give it a genuine shot. It almost sounded like a challenge and the competitor in me got fired up. I told myself I would make a game out of it and eat nothing but good clean wholesome food. At the end of the 30 days I would evaluate how I felt and see if this new lifestyle was for me. Long story short, over that month I dove in to learning about different foods and how our bodies consume food for energy. I learned about micronutrients, macronutrients, digestive enzymes, and a whole lot more.

Each day I evaluated how I felt and stuck to my new lifestyle change without wavering. As the days went by I noticed my energy levels started to increase, I was sleeping better, my skin looked clearer, my mind seemed to remember things easier, and I even had a more positive outlook on life. It was at that moment I knew this lifestyle change was here to stay.

Over the last 7 years I have refined my diet to eating what's called the Paleo diet (or caveman diet), which consists of protein intake from animals, healthy fats, and a ton of carbs from fruits and vegetables. Yes, you heard me right. I eat a ton of carbs! The trick is to eat the *right* types of carbs and I explain all of this a little later in the book. I have never felt better and I'm never going back to my old ways... EVER!

My intention with this book is to show you how to live a life of health and vitality, that is filled with energy each and every day without thinking too much about your diet, calories, fat intake, and other mind-consuming pointless tasks.

I want to do something a little different with this book. I talk to people all the time about their different "diets" and what they think will work, but at the end of the day, the Paleo lifestyle is one that continues to work for people all over the world.

I want to show you that it isn't complicated to stick to a healthy lifestyle - and that's exactly what you will learn by reading this book. It's not about a diet, fad, magic pill, program or gimmick. Like I've said, it's about a way of life, and you have to understand that first before we start this journey together. I'm designing this book to be an easy read without a lot of the technical talk, because I feel that if I overload you with a ton of information, it is going to overwhelm you and you're never going to get on the right track. So, I condensed this book down and made it extremely easy to digest and absorb all the necessary information you need to start this new lifestyle and get your health and life back on track.

Important

It is important to know that this book could have been well over 300 pages if I wanted to pad it with fluffy stories and hard-to-understand medical concepts. I decided to strip it all out and give you the basics of this diet. I chose to not cover all of the science and facts pertaining to Paleo diet research within the body of this book (for those of you who want the research, I have included a few links in the back of the book). There is a ton of data and facts out there and it's easily accessible.

Instead, I want to give you everything I've researched and found to be true, as well as the necessary knowledge to go forward with your own experimentation of the Paleo lifestyle. This way, you can see if this diet is for you. I don't hold to the belief that the Paleo diet is for every single person on earth, or that you have to stick to the Paleo diet or you won't be able to lose weight. In fact, I suggest that it is a good thing to give yourself cheat days with wiggle room every now and then. It is good to stick to a 90/10 ratio - meaning, eat healthy and stick to the Paleo plan 90% of the time and the other 10% can be wiggle room for cheat days and small indulgences here and there. This is something that goes against the grain of many other Paleo books, but like I said, I think about things a little differently from most people.

Read through the book, try it, see how you feel, and evaluate your daily life and make adjustments accordingly. Every one of us is different and we all respond to foods and diets differently - bottom line - give it a shot and see how you feel, because at the end of the day, that's the only real science you need.

Our diet and health should never be a constant thought in our mind. We eat to survive, and food is fuel for the body. Back in the days of our ancient ancestors, they didn't think about calories and fat content. The word "carbs" never came into their conversations and yet they lived an extremely healthy and fit lifestyle, and were able to have the energy necessary to hunt and gather food each and every day. Why is this the case? Why do you have to think so much about your daily caloric intake? It isn't about that. I want you to get 'counting calories' out of your mind right now.

Once you fully grasp the idea of the Paleo lifestyle, you'll begin to see that this way of life has far more benefits than the typical American diet has to offer. The Paleo lifestyle can help reverse diabetes, slow depression, help with G.I. problems, and help your immune system reach its peak potential!

Understanding The Basics Of The Paleo Diet

In order to fully understand how this lifestyle change is going to help you in the long run, it is essential that you understand the basic core components of the foods you eat. However, before we get to that I want to be real with you for a minute.

The Paleo diet is a lifestyle change and you have to understand that RIGHT NOW. I know all too well how easy it is to stop for fast food or microwave one of those frozen dinners because I used to do it A LOT. You are better than that and you can give this diet change an honest shot. You owe it to your family and friends, but more importantly, you owe it to yourself.

I also want to address the term "Paleo" for a second. The word "paleo" is just a word to describe a way of eating a natural clean diet. I know a lot of people that get too caught up in the concept of cavemen running around hunting and gathering food all day. I often have people dissecting little facets of the diet and scrutinizing every detail and that is not what it's about. We live in a modern age, which means we have better technology and resources than our ancient ancestors ever did. We are simply borrowing concepts and food sources from our predecessors and bringing that knowledge to the modern age.

Now, I promise that I'll make this as interesting as possible, but it is important that you really understand these parts because this is what's going to make up the core of your diet. We're going to start off with one of my favorite groups: proteins.

Proteins

Proteins are the building blocks of life. They make up our skin, muscle, hair, and nails, among other things, and they interact with a bunch of different parts of our body such as our neurotransmitters, enzymes, and hormones. The truth is, you can find protein in a lot of different sources, but I like to categorize these into two areas: top-shelf protein and bottom-shelf protein. Top-shelf proteins are proteins that you get from food such as fish, chicken, beef, eggs, and shellfish. Bottom-shelf proteins are proteins such as nuts, beans, and rice. This is one misconception that a lot of people have when studying different nutrition plans. These bottom shelf proteins will keep you alive and they will give you nutrition, but it will not be the core and foundation of your new Paleo lifestyle. The most important aspect of protein that we need to take into consideration is the fact that they're made up of molecules called amino acids. We need amino acids because they are essential to our survival and they are the building blocks of human life. I want you to keep this in mind as you read the rest of this book.

Carbohydrates a.k.a. Carbs

If you're an Olympic athlete, carbohydrates are an essential part of your diet. If you're a weightlifter or bodybuilder, carbohydrates can also be an essential part of your diet. The problem, however, is that society has defined carbohydrates in such a way that gives them a bad reputation, when in fact they are an essential part of our diet - when used in the right manner. That last bit is key because carbohydrates can be broken down into two separate groups (like proteins).

Without getting too technical on you, we have monosaccharides and disaccharides. "Mono" simply means one sugar and "di" simply means two sugars. This is why we are going to concentrate on the carbohydrates that will actually help your body improve energy levels and help your digestive system at the same time.

Let me be clear about one thing - the Paleo diet is not a "low carb" diet by any means. In fact the

Paleo diet could be categorized as a high carb diet if you wanted to look at it that way. We just have to look at carbs in a different way and get them from the right sources (Mostly vegetables and some fruit). I'll be going over this shortly, but for now just remember that we aren't cutting carbs here, we're just getting them from the right sources. :) We'll get into the different types of carbs in a little bit.

Fats

This is the part of the Paleo lifestyle that people often misunderstand and sometimes get upset about. That's only because we are conditioned to think that fat is a bad thing. But the truth is, we need certain types of fat in our diet to keep us at our optimal energy levels. Again, we will go over the different types of fats that will make your life amazing a little later on.

Insulin

One of the biggest causes of fat storage has to do with the hormone we call insulin. You may have heard the term 'insulin' thrown around before on TV or read about it on the Internet - and there's a good reason for it. Insulin is critical in regulating your blood sugar levels, your body fat, and also deals with aging factors. To live a long and vibrant life, we need to do our best to keep our insulin levels on the low side by controlling the foods we put in our body - specifically, carbohydrates that tend to spike insulin and cause our bodies to store fat.

To understand insulin, we have to also look at insulin's role in regulating our blood sugar levels. Insulin's primary role is to tell the nutrients you put into your body where to be stored. If you are constantly putting high carbohydrate (bad carbs - bread, pasta, etc.) meals and sugary foods into your system, your insulin levels spike and your body tells itself to store that energy as fat. This is why the Paleo lifestyle avoids such foods and allows your body to process itself and regulate insulin levels efficiently.

Let's talk about GRAINS!

When you make the jump and decide to try Paleo, or dive in full-time, it is important that you understand the one essential ingredient you need to eliminate from your diet - Grains. Grains include everything from Barley wheat, corn, oats, rice and so on. However, as comfortable as you are eating these things, it is important to know that grains are far less nutritious than normal vegetables, fruits, nuts, and proteins.

Grains have a reputation for stimulating improper liver, thyroid, and pancreas responses in many people which can, in turn, lead to a reduced immune system, fungal infections, skin problems, anxiety, depression and weight gain. One of the problems about grains is that they inhibit the body from proper digestion. This goes back to the way grains evolved as a plant species. They essentially grow with no defense mechanism and our bodies just aren't adapted to digest these types of grains - period.

One term that is been thrown around lately is the term 'gluten.' Gluten comes from the latin word for "glue" which is the first clue that this ingredient shouldn't be put into the human body. Gluten is a type of protein that is found in wheat, rye oats, and barley, and it is the ingredient that helps dough rise and gives pasta its bouncy consistency. We aren't going to dive deep into what gluten is, but I want you to know it isn't good for any of us, and it's important to eliminate it from your diet.

I'm not going to beat around the bush... whether you want to hear it or not, grains are not that healthy for you. I know, I said it! All these foods taste good. The bread, pastas, cookies, you name it – they are all extremely delicious - but you have to look past your taste buds for one second in order to get to the real truth of the matter, and to understand what foods will actually help you live and not kill you. Let's dive in to the anatomy of a grain to really understand it.

All grains are comprised of three parts: endosperm, bran, and germ. If that sounds weird, just bear with me for a minute here. Like I said, I'm giving you the nuts and bolts of the boring stuff so that you can understand the Paleo diet and have enough info to make a decision about whether it is the right lifestyle for you. I believe everyone can benefit from eating Paleo, but this is ultimately something you have to try for yourself and gauge how well you feel. Ok, back to grains:

Bran

Bran is the outer covering of a whole, unprocessed grain. It contains some vitamins, minerals, and a host of other proteins and anti-nutrients designed to prevent the predation, or eating of the grain.

Endosperm

The endosperm is a starch with a little bit of protein. This is the energy supply of a growing grain embryo.

Germ

The germ (sometimes referred to as cereal germ) is the portion of the grain that acts as its reproductive system. In nature, the cereal grain is distributed by the wind, and when everything falls into place, the embryo begins the process of growth using the endosperm for energy. This is the place where vegetable oil typically derives from.

A Note About Oats

I understand that there are a lot of people out there who love to eat their morning oatmeal. But I have some bad news… oatmeal contains several proteins similar to gluten. These proteins are hard to digest, and thus remain intact despite the best efforts of the digestive process to break them down. Kind of a bummer, right? Well, let me just put it this way… try your best to go without any type of grains for 30 days and see how you feel. I guarantee that you'll notice a major difference in the way your digestive system, your energy levels and your overall health and vitality work. I want you to get the term "whole-grain" out of your head for the duration of this experiment. This is a term used by companies to get us to think that whole grains are a healthy substitute for natural foods.

When you compare grains calorie-for-calorie to other natural foods such as lean meats, seafood, and veggies, you understand that they are a far weaker type of calorie and not suitable for sustained energy. This also means that you can't eat stuff like quinoa as well. I know a lot of people out there have found quinoa (pronounced KEEN-WAH) to be an alternative to whole-grains, but those don't fly either. Because they are in the same family as grains, they still have the same type of side effects on the digestive system as grains.

The biggest issue you have to worry about is the havoc they wreak on your digestive system. They tend to cause what's called malabsorption which, in turn, affects your health and well-being. Let's go over a few of the issues related to trying to absorb grains in your diet:

For starters, grains have the tendency to damage the lining of the gut. When the gut is damaged, your ability to absorb nutrients is greatly diminished. We need the healthy lining of our stomach to absorb all the nutrients we need for our bodies. This includes all proteins, fats, carbs, vitamins and minerals.

There is also the risk for the gall bladder to be damaged. This will inhibit the production of bile, which means we will not be able to absorb essential nutrients such as vitamins A, D, and K. If you can't absorb these vitamins, you're going to have to figure out alternative ways to get them into your body. Trust me, you want to get these vitamins from food!

Once your gut lining goes, it opens the door for autoimmunity deficiencies and cancer. Not Good. The pancreas is especially affected by inflammation caused by grains passing through. This can cause pancreatic cancer or inflammation of the pancreas.

> *Bottom line is this... grains aren't meant for the body and can cause digestive system problems, which can lead to more serious problems such as multiple sclerosis, rheumatoid arthritis, lupus, vitiligo, narcolepsy, autism, and a variety of other diseases.

Now, I know you may be saying, "But, I don't have any of these diseases!" I know, but you have to understand that over time, these are the issues that arise when we don't take care of our bodies and efficiently fuel them with the right nutrients and whole foods.

A Word About Beans And Dairy

Several diets in today's diet world have incorporated the use of beans (or legumes) as a healthy substitute for carbohydrates and proteins within your diet. Beans aren't necessarily evil, but they do lead to similar problems as grains. Gut irritation, anti-nutrients, as well as inflammation. I do eat black beans from time to time if I feel like I am not getting enough carbs from my fruits and veggies, but for your 30 day experiment, leave them out.

Fat

Fat seems to be one of the most confusing aspects of the Paleo diet today - and for good reason. Ever since the FDA got involved in the food process, we've been told that fat is a bad thing. This may be for good reason but we have to think of fat as an added value to each and every meal we eat. The general population doesn't have a hard time understanding that carbs are not good for you, but when it comes to fat, we are in the dark most the time.

The funny thing about fat is our bodies are made up of a lot of it. This includes our organs, brain, nerves, and even reproductive hormones. But to accurately understand how fat helps the body, you have to understand the subtypes of fats. There are three types of fats: saturated, monounsaturated, and polyunsaturated. You don't have to understand everything about the science behind it, but it is good to understand the basics so you're not in the dark.

Monounsaturated Fats

This type of fat is commonly referred to as oleic acid and is found mainly in foods such as avocado, olive oil, and nuts (almonds, walnuts, etc.). This type of fat is also found in grass-fed beef, which happens to be one of the staples of the Paleo diet. These fats are actually quite amazing, as they tend to help improve insulin sensitivity, improve glucagon response, and decrease cholesterol levels.

Polyunsaturated Fats

While monounsaturated fats are typically considered a healthier type of fat, polyunsaturated fatty acids are better for you than saturated fatty acids. This is because they are known to reduce bad cholesterol (LDL) and increase good cholesterol (HDL). Polyunsaturated fats also contain essential fatty acids like Omega-3 and Omega-6. These are fatty acids that the body needs, but cannot necessarily produce on its own. These types of fats are also important because they send a signal to your brain to let you know when you are full. This will prevent overeating and can also help you lose weight. Bottom line, polyunsaturated fats are important.

Cut The Trans Fats!

Let's just say that trans fats aren't the best thing for you, but I'm sure you've heard others mention this. Trans fats are created when polyunsaturated fats from foods such as corn and soybeans, are exposed to heat. The resulting fats look similar to saturated fats. They have a reputation of ruining liver function and destroying insulin sensitivity.

The Omegas (Omega-3 and Omega-6)

These types of fats are important as they help deal with inflammation in the body, and are known to help control various cancer elements (typically in anything that is related to inflammation issues).

Omega-3 fatty acids are categorized as anti-inflammatory, while Omega-6 are categorized as pro-inflammatory. The goal with our nutrition should be to even the ratio between these two Omegas. Most people are lacking in Omega-3, which can be satisfied with foods such as wild fish, grass-fed beef, and some egg sources.

Omega-3 can also be taken in supplement form, but try to minimize the use of supplements as much as possible when trying to stick to a Paleo diet. I'll touch on supplements a little later.

List of Omega-3 Foods You Should Be Eating:

- Wild salmon
- Anchovies
- Mackerel
- Herring
- Trout
- Omega-3 Eggs (my favorite)
- Grass-Fed Natural Beef
- An assortment of nuts and seeds (walnuts and flaxseed, for example)

So, You Like To Party, Huh? (Alcohol and Paleo)

Before I say anything, I want you to know that alcohol is not part of the Paleo diet, but it is a part of our social culture and it is one area where you can bend the rules a little (if you so choose).

I'll be the first to admit that I like to have a good time, but with that said, I ALWAYS value my health way above any good night out. I know I know...I hear you saying it now, "But, no one wants to be the buzz kill of the party!" Yes, I agree, and lucky for all of us, we can still have a good time and be "healthier" if we take some time and think about it before-hand.

Here are some rules to live by before you go out:

- Always do most of your heavier drinking earlier in the night.
- Stay away from sugary drinks (you know, the pina coladas, jack and cokes, etc.)
- No soda (besides club soda)
- Stick to clear liquor (preferably tequila)

- Don't mix alcohol (especially hard alcohol with beer)
- Try to eat a high protein meal after you drink

Here is a drink recipe I stick to when I go out:

- 1-2 shots of tequila or vodka
- A whole lime or lemon (I like a lot)
- Soda water

This is a drink that will give you the kick you seek without the crazy sugar intake and (hopefully) without the morning headache.

You don't want to be the "Debbie Downer" of the party, and if you stick to drinks similar to this, you'll fit right in and still enjoy yourself. :)

A Word about Beer and Wine

I do enjoy a good beer, but I only drink it socially and tend to stick to craft beer when I do drink it. Stick to dry red wine if you have to choose, as it has less sugar and has been known to aid in sports recovery due to resveratrol (aids in inflammation reduction).

The Paleo Diet and Exercise

I know this isn't a workout book, but I think it is important to discuss fitness when dealing with your new lifestyle on the Paleo diet. Working out and being active, in general, has become one of the most profitable industries in the world. Why is it then that we have so many obese people in our country who don't take their health and fitness seriously?

I want to show you that working out doesn't have to be a time or mind-consuming activity. In fact, I work out less than three hours per week (and I know others who do the same), and I am in great shape and have energy to spare. This is all possible because of my Paleo diet lifestyle. So what does this mean? This means that you don't have to spend your life in a gym wasting time pumping weights and running on the treadmill! Yay!

In my personal life, I've boiled down working out into the smallest amount of work possible for the most results possible. Let me explain this concept really fast. When you work out 6 days a week for one or two hours a day, your body does not have the necessary time to recuperate and regenerate your muscles properly. We as human beings were designed, and have evolved, to need periods of rest where our bodies can rebuild itself in preparation for the next day's tasks.

Our ancient ancestors didn't have cars or grocery stores or any of the luxuries we have today; therefore, they had to be in good physical health in order to do the routine things in life - like travel, hunt and gather food. Think about it, if you couldn't hunt and gather food and be physically active and walk around, how were you going to survive? That is why it is important to understand that physical fitness plays a big role in your happiness and your life abundance.

Working Out Doesn't Have To Be Tedious

Working out doesn't have to be hard or time-consuming. I would suggest that you start out with easy exercises with the goal of activating your muscles to a point where your heart starts to beat and pump blood through your system.

This can be as easy as doing a set of 15 to 20 push-ups, or 30 to 40 air squats and light to moderate walking.

Here is a sample weekly workout routine that is easy, not time-consuming, and will leave you feeling energized.

Daily Workout Routine:

- Monday: 15-20 push-ups* and 30 air squats upon waking
- Tuesday: 30 air squats upon waking and going to bed
- Wednesday: 15 push-ups* and 30 air squats upon waking
- Thursday: 30 air squats upon waking and going to bed
- Friday: 15-20 push-ups* and 30 air squats upon waking
- Saturday: 30 air squats upon waking and going to bed
- Sunday: REST

I would also recommend walking to moderate jogging 3 times a week or more. This does not mean you have to run 1+ miles per day, but it is important to get out and be active. If you are starting to feel lethargic at any point throughout the day (at work or around the house), get up and go to a secluded place (i.e. bathroom) and do 20 to 30 air squats. It will get your heart pumping and give you a slight energy boost.

*If you can't do regular pushups yet, that's ok. Just use your knees on the floor, or do standing push-ups against the wall (you literally stand about 2 feet from the wall and do a push-up as if you're on the floor).

As you can see, this routine is very simple and might take a total of 30 minutes per week - IF that. You won't necessarily feel sore, unless you really don't exercise at all, but this simple short routine can help jumpstart you into a more active lifestyle and can help your heart stay healthy. From there, you can always build upon this routine and up your repetitions or even add weights into the mix.

Note: An easy place to do air squats is in the shower if it's big enough. It takes literally 1 to 2 minutes and it really jump starts your day.

Integrating The Paleo Diet Into Your Life

Okay, so we've gone over what the Paleo diet is and how it works, but now it's time to implement the Paleo diet into your everyday life. This is where the rubber hits the road. People often ask me about my diet - They'll ask, "You look good, what do you eat?" At this point I smile and begin to explain how I eat, and how the Paleo diet has changed my eating habits for good.

The beauty of the Paleo diet lies in its simplicity. I don't know about you, but I don't really want to worry about what to eat, when to eat, etc. The Paleo diet gives you the flexibility to take your mind and cravings out of the equation. It's amazing because it's minimalistic at its core, which allows you to focus on your life and not your food intake.

The Paleo diet does't have to be hard. In fact, the Paleo lifestyle allows you to eat when (and if) you need to eat. Let me explain... with some diets, you might be given a specific eating plan with certain times to eat with certain types of food to eat. This is where the Paleo lifestyle is different. When you're eating Paleo, you simply eat when you're hungry. What an amazing concept! When your body needs fuel it will let you know (usually through hunger pangs). Then you fuel up with the right nutrient dense foods we've been talking about and back to your day you go. Really simple here, folks.

Like I mentioned before, I want you to try this "lifestyle" for 30 days. After 30 days, you will know if this is something you will want to stick to. And really, with everything in life, that's how it should be. As long as what you're doing isn't harmful to you, it's okay to try different things and see if it works for your body. However, I have a sneaking suspicion that you will be pleasantly surprised with the results of sticking to the Paleo diet.

Benefits of the Paleo diet as described by others and myself:

- You get to eat all the food you want, as long as it's Paleo-compliant
- You don't have to worry about fat intake
- You don't have to count calories
- It reduces bloating
- Your skin gets clearer and more vibrant
- You feel stronger

- You lose fat and gain muscle (or keep muscle you have)
- Your grocery shopping time is drastically reduced
- Improves blood pressure and decreases insulin secretion, which allows weight-loss to occur.

It's Time For A Kitchen Audit!

We're about to take this Paleo journey to my favorite destination - the grocery store - but before we get there we have a very important task to complete. I call this the kitchen audit.

Before you make your first grocery trip, I want you to go through your pantry and cupboards and take out all of the food you know is not Paleo.

This includes:

- cereal
- bread
- sugary foods
- cookies
- ice cream
- frozen pizzas
- anything processed
- soda
- juices from concentrate
- snacks (crackers, girl scout cookies, etc.)

- anything you know in your heart that is not good for you
- dairy products (milk, yogurt, sour cream, cheese etc.)

Things you can keep:

- any meat (poultry, fish, beef, etc.)
- vegetables
- fruit
- packaged lunch meats are ok
- nuts
- tea
- coffee

I want you to start with a clean slate and this is the best way to do it. You may be saying, "I bought all of that stuff!" Yes you're right. The way I see it you have 3 options:

Option 1 - Start your Paleo diet once all of the "bad stuff" in your house is consumed (not my favorite option).

Option 2 - Throw it all in the trash and start fresh.

Option 3 - Drive all of this food to a food bank or homeless shelter and teach your kids (if you have kids) a lesson about helping those less fortunate.

If it were me, I would start right away while you're excited to give this Paleo stuff a shot. You're going to feel liberated after this task, knowing that you are taking your health into your own hands and making a change that will improve your life for the better!

First stop... Grocery store

When starting the Paleo diet, it is essential that you completely forego and throw out your old mentality of buying groceries. I am sure you've heard this before, but you want to stick to the perimeter of the grocery store – not the freezer section, not the bread section, not the dessert section, but the sections that include meats and produce.

Produce

Let's start with the produce section first. You want to load up on as many veggies as you possibly can. This means you can go absolutely nuts with the types of vegetables you want to buy. I typically eat a ton of broccoli, carrots, squash, cauliflower, spinach and kale. You can buy fruit as well (and you should), but I would recommend having a ratio of 3:1 (veggies to fruits) when starting out on the Paleo diet. This is because you want to limit the amount of sugar you are taking in at first, and fruits contain a lot of sugar even though they are healthy and provide antioxidants and other nutritional benefits.

I can't emphasize this enough... vegetables are super fuel for our bodies. If you don't like vegetables, please train yourself to love them. A few years back I wasn't too fond of veggies, but now I couldn't live without them. There are ways to prepare them that make them tasty - whether you bake them, sauté them, steam them or eat them raw, find a way to cook them that appeals to you and stick to it.

A Word About Organic

"Organic" is a very highly-debated topic in today's health world. Should you buy organic or not? I typically don't buy everything organic because, quite frankly, you don't have to. I typically stick to the few items that I know are treated with pesticides and chemicals, and those items I will buy organic.

A few items that I always buy organic:

- Peppers
- Peaches
- Apples
- Nectarines
- Strawberries
- Cherries
- Grapes
- Spinach
- Celery
- Kale
- Lettuce

A few items that are okay to buy non-organic (these foods typically don't absorb pesticides, or have outer skin that protects them from pesticides):

• Asparagus
• Avocados
• Bananas
• Broccoli
• Cabbage
• Kiwi
• Mango
• Onions
• Papaya
• Pineapple

Meat/Poultry

This section is easy, especially if you like protein! There really aren't any rules when it comes to meats except, try to stick to leaner cuts of conventional meats such as pork loin, lean ground beef (I try to buy 93/7), chicken breasts, turkey breast, etc..

When buying any type of beef, a.k.a. steak, bison or anything similar, it is always best to buy grass-fed because this will alter the Omega-3 and Omega-6 fat ratios in the meat. Typically what happens is that most large-production volume dairies and farms feed their animals a diet consisting of grains. This tends to make animals fat and bloated and, like we mentioned before, throws off the Omega fat ratios.

Bison is actually one of my favorite meats because it is high in protein and extremely lean. If you've never tried it, I suggest you give it a whirl. You might be pleasantly surprised.

Seafood

If you don't like seafood, I would suggest trying a few new varieties to see if you can adapt your taste buds. Fish and other types of seafood, such as shrimp, are extremely beneficial to your health and provide a ton of nutrients such as healthy Omega-3 fats.

I typically stick to wild fish such as salmon from Alaska, and shellfish such as shrimp and mussels. Tilapia is also a great choice because it is extremely low in fat and high in protein. You won't feel bloated and you'll be able to digest this type of fish extremely easily.

Eggs

I'm going to start off this little bit by saying that some days I eat over 10 eggs (I eat eggs everyday but the number fluctuates depending on my mood). Yikes! You may think that sounds crazy, but I can assure you it is not. There are so many misconceptions and misinformation floating around about eggs, that I want to do my best to dispel some of those myths right now.

Eggs are one of the most wholesome and nutritious, complete foods you can eat, and it just so happens that they are extremely cheap as well! The cool thing about eggs is that they help you burn fat more efficiently and also have a high-protein count, to boot. I would suggest, however, that you stick to Omega-3 enriched eggs. You'll find that these types of eggs are always labeled with high Omega-3 labels.

The only thing you have to worry about is autoimmune conditions – if you suffer from an autoimmune condition, try eating a few eggs a day to see how you feel. If you feel okay, go ahead and continue making eggs part of your everyday diet.

Your Paleo Grocery List

So you've read through the last section and now you're wondering what to buy at the grocery store. Well, I like to keep things simple, so we will start with the basics and then build from there. The following is a breakdown of items you should buy. Once you get the gist of it, you can get a little more creative.

My Paleo Essentials (not in any particular order)

I want to start with my essentials list and then break down the main categories in-depth after that. I do eat the majority of things on this shopping list, but I have found these items are the easiest to prepare and consume. The following are my go-to items that I always have stocked up:

- Chicken breast (boneless, skinless)
- Grass-fed beef (or I get my beef intake from Chipotle - discussed a little later)
- Salmon (frozen filets work fine)
- Tilapia (frozen filets work fine)
- Almonds
- Cashew and Almond butter
- Almond and Coconut milk

- Coconut water (gets pricey but it's very good for you)
- Apples and grapefruit (My go-to fruit choices)
- Broccoli (I like fresh but I will typically buy the pre packaged, ready to steam variety from Whole Foods or Trader Joe's type markets)
- Kale and Spinach
- Olive Oil and Coconut Oil (Cook everything with this and use it on salads)
- Avocados (These are a must. They do tend to be pricey, but look in places like Walmart where you can find them for 64 cents a piece)
- 85% or 90% dark chocolate (for sugar cravings)

Oils (Healthy fats)

Healthy oils such as olive oil and coconut oil are some of the best healthy fats out there. These are two ingredients that I truly can't live without. Olive oil is my go-to and I almost never cook a meal without it.

Baking chicken? Drizzle it on top before you put it in the oven. Scrambling eggs? Coat the pan with it before you put the eggs in. Try to stick to organic if possible or better name brands if possible.

- Olive oil
- Coconut oil

Meat

Grass-fed beef is king and I would splurge a little here if possible. Excellent source of protein and healthy fats.

- Chicken
- Grass-fed beef
- Pork tenderloin
- Lean ground beef (I look for 93/7 or 85/15 - fat content)
- Lean ground turkey (I look for 99/1 - fat content)

Seafood:
As with anything, fresh is almost always better, BUT I do realize some people are on a budget and that is totally understandable. Fresh seafood is pricey, but if you can afford it, go fresh. Personally, I will mix it up with fresh when I can, but frozen seafood is very convenient (lasts a while) and I eat that too.
(TIP - Walmart Superstores and other stores, such as Costco, have a pretty good deal on large bags of tilapia and salmon filets. Just thaw before preparing and you're good to go)

- Shrimp (fresh or frozen)
- Tilapia (fresh or frozen filets)
- Atlantic wild salmon (fresh or frozen filets)
- Catfish

• Most fish types will be fine

Vegetables

This is a no brainer... you can go absolutely hog wild (is that a phrase?) with vegetables. Try and stick to leafy greens because they are your best friend.

• Broccoli
• Cauliflower
• Asparagus
• Spinach
• Kale
• Cucumbers
• Squash/zucchini
• Sweet potatoes
• Any leafy green vegetable

TIP - You can eat pretty much any vegetable you want - I would stick to the most common and cheaper varieties to start.

A Word about Fruit

I want to address fruit for a second because it's kind of a big deal. Yes fruit is healthy and it can benefit you immensely. However, when you first start the Paleo lifestyle, I would suggest and recommend not eating fruit as frequently as you might be doing now. Fruit has a high sugar level, which could lead to insulin spikes, which will in turn cause fat storage in your body. I would recommend eating mainly vegetables to start, and incorporate fruit here and there.

For example, eating grapefruit in the morning is a metabolism booster and blueberries have a lot of antioxidants. So, it is true that fruits are very healthy, but I will once again reference the 90/10 rule - 90% of your carbohydrate intake should be vegetable-based and 10% should be fruit-based. Also, you want to eat fruit earlier in the day, if possible, preferably with breakfast. This will give you energy for your daily routine, and help avoid insulin spikes at night while you sleep.

Fresh Fruits

- Grapefruit
- Oranges
- Lemon
- Lime
- Blueberries
- Strawberries
- Raspberries
- BlackBerries
- Cranberries
- Apricots
- Peaches

- Nectarines
- Cherries
- Melon
- Apple
- Pears
- Mango
- Kiwi
- Coconut
- Pineapple

Eggs

Omega-3 enriched and/or organic are great. Eggs are cheap and a great food to have for snacks or even a meal. Hard boil eggs for those times when you need a quick healthy snack. Eggs are underrated! Don't be afraid of them.

Beverages

Beverages aren't that complicated, but I do understand how addicting soda is (I used to be addicted to the stuff). STAY AWAY from soda at all costs. It is EVIL (tell yourself this every time you have a craving). Pure filtered water is best, but you can drink other beverages, including:

- Water (filtered)
- Coconut water (unsweetened)
- Black coffee or espresso (NO sugary lattes or fancy drinks!)

- Natural Teas (Green Tea, Yerba Mate , etc.)
- Juiced vegetables and fruit (SEE BELOW)
- Almond Milk
- Coconut Milk - this stuff is great

Note - I would buy a lot of lemons to add to your water. Tastes great and they are extremely good for you.

Juicing

I believe whole-heartedly in 2 things: the Paleo Diet and Juicing. Juicing is something that I STRONGLY recommend doing, especially when you're on the Paleo diet. Some might think, "Did our ancient ancestors juice fruits and vegetables?" Obviously not, but we might as well use this technology to further our diet. I would strongly recommend juicing in conjunction with your new Paleo lifestyle.

It's an amazing habit to form, and it will leave you feeling rejuvenated and energized. This isn't a book on juicing, but if you would like to know more about juicing for weight loss and energy, you can check out my other book where I explain in detail how you can incorporate juicing into your everyday life. It's currently on sale and extremely cheap.

Visit---> **FCRW.org/juicing**

Nuts and Seeds

Nuts and seeds are an essential part of the Paleo lifestyle. They provide healthy fat and are able to be consumed rather easily. Keep nuts in the car or in the office for whenever you are feeling a little hungry. Eat a few here and a few there, but don't go "nuts" (pun intended). Too much of a good thing can be a bad thing.

• Raw almonds
• Cashews
• Macadamia nuts
• Pistachios
• Walnuts

A Word about Peanuts

I do love peanuts, however, peanuts are technically considered a legume and should not be eaten on the Paleo diet. They are a common food allergen and do more damage than good. Just avoid them during your 30 day paleo trial. At the end of 30 days, see how you feel. If you want to test peanuts in your diet, go for it.

Spices

This is an area where you can spice it up (pun intended) anyway you want. Here's a list of common spices you can use. These will get you started. You can use a variety of others if you wish.

- Pepper
- Sea Salt
- Garlic Salt
- Lemon Pepper
- Cumin
- Nutmeg
- Cinnamon
- Paprika

Herbs

Herbs are similar to spices. You can mix-and-match whatever you want to your liking.

- Cilantro
- Rosemary
- Thyme
- Basil

Taking Care of Cravings (Treats)

Sometimes when you get a sweet tooth it is good to have something around the house you can munch on to curb your sweet appetite. I typically keep dark chocolate lying around - usually 80 to 90% Cacao. Cacao is actually a strong antioxidant in its raw form, and if you're going to eat something sweet, dark chocolate is a good way to go.

I would also suggest eating fruit, as this tends to curb sugar cravings. Cut up an orange or an apple and see how you feel after that. I don't like to recommend a ton of fruit at first, because fruit can tend to spike insulin levels as you've already learned.

• Raw honey
• Hundred percent maple syrup
• Gluten-free flour (such as coconut)
• Raw milk

I've also added some dessert recipes to the back of the book, which you may find to be quite tasty.

Eating Out Paleo Style

Eating out is one of those fun things that we all enjoy and love to do. It's great having someone cook for you and bring you food without having to do any work yourself. Just be careful when you go out to eat, because these places are not your best friend when it comes to your new Paleo lifestyle. There are, however, things you can eat at pretty much any restaurant that will allow you to stick to your lifestyle and new eating plan.

Below is a list of restaurants where you can eat and still be on the Paleo diet. Remember that it's okay to cheat every now and then, and when I say 'cheat,' I mean things like a slice of cheese here and there isn't going to kill you. A little bit of dressing or sauce isn't going to kill you either. Just be conscious of when you're making these 'cheat' decisions, and try not to make them too often. Life is meant to be enjoyed, and you don't have to be a hundred percent strict every step of the way. Like I said in the beginning of this book, if you can stick to a 90/10 ratio, you'll be fine.

Chipotle (or similar fast casual restaurant)

I'm going to come right out and say it - I love Chipotle. It's one of those restaurants where I can eat every day because it's similar to the way I cook for myself at home. I can go out, eat a healthy delicious meal, and not feel guilty about it. I also appreciate that Chipotle makes it known that they use fresh ingredients. I typically get my beef from Chipotle because it tastes great and is a little less expensive than buying it in the grocery store.

What I get:
I typically get a burrito bowl with no rice, a little black beans, extra fajitas, and veggies with double meat. I'll top this off with three of the salsas and lettuce, and that's it. It's tasty, delicious, and I feel great after eating it. As you might've noticed, I don't get any sour cream or cheese. And definitely no tortillas! Guacamole is ok too, but I'm not exactly sure what they put in it so you're on your own with that one.

In-N-Out Burger (or any burger joint that offers lettuce wrapped burgers)

I even eat at In-N-Out burger sometimes (if you're on the West Coast, you know what I'm talking about). This actually goes for any burger joint that will serve you what's called "protein" or "lettuce style." Just have them wrap the burger and everything inside it with lettuce, and you're good to go!

What I Get:
Double Single (2 meats, 1 cheese - I cheat a little there), extra tomatoes, pickles, both kinds of onions - raw and grilled, light spread.

Thai Food

I love Thai food and I love it especially because it fits within the Paleo lifestyle guidelines. Typically, curries and cashew chicken are great choices. Just remember to cut out the rice.

What I Get:
Typically I will get cashew chicken, some type of curry, and a large side of vegetables, with green tea. NO RICE!

Woodranch (or a BBQ-style restaurant)

BBQ-style restaurants are typically considered "unhealthy," but this has more to do with buttered biscuits, mashed potatoes, mac & cheese, etc. If you stick to the proteins and vegetables, you'll be golden.

What I get:
When I go out to these types of restaurants, I typically like to get beef as a treat to myself. I'll stick to prime rib or tri-tip, but any steak will do. Chicken is also a great option, but it's easily-available at markets, so go wild and try something new. I'll then get a ton of vegetables (no butter) and chow down.

Sushi

Sushi is great, but when I talk about sushi I mean sashimi, specifically. You know, the raw fish that is delicately-sliced, and prepared neatly on your plate. If you stick to this type of fish, it is delicious and it is high in protein.

What I get:
I tend to stick to high-caliber-grade sashimi such as albacore, salmon, tuna, and eel. I will also ask for a side of avocado and a side of vegetables as well. This way I get all of my fats, proteins, and carbs in one delicious meal. Miso soup is also great.

Seafood Restaurants

Seafood restaurants are really easy because most seafood is okay to eat. As you can imagine, eating in a seafood restaurant is pretty straightforward. Stick to the healthy fatty fishes and vegetables, and you're golden.

What I get:
I tend to stick to salmon, vegetables, and avocado if they have it.

Are you seeing a trend here? It's pretty obvious that this lifestyle isn't that complicated, and you can eat out just about anywhere. Just stick to the three main food groups (Fats, proteins, carbohydrates from veggies) and you'll still be able to enjoy a nice evening out with delicious food prepared for you without having to cook.

Always Be Stocked Up

The number one failure point that I tend to see is when people run out of their Paleo food stock. When you run out of the foods you should be eating, it is extremely easy to slip and fall back to whatever you have lying around your kitchen, pantry, or refrigerator.

If you run out of your Paleo food, most likely you'll be too lazy to go to the store to restock. This is when temptation sets in and you start eating things like chips and cookies or whatever's lying around your house (hopefully you've done the kitchen audit already!).

This is why stocking up with the right foods and being on top of your shopping is an essential part of living the Paleo lifestyle. Just like our ancient ancestors had to plan ahead and hunt and forage for food, we have to do the same and go to the grocery store to keep fuel (i.e., food) ready to go.

Supplements on The Paleo Diet

Oh, the old supplement question. I get this often because we have been force-fed so many advertisements about which supplements will make us bigger, faster, and stronger. I personally used to take a lot of supplements until I realized that they really only help 10%, if that. And most don't do much at all. I do, however, recommend a few supplements that will help you. They are listed as follows:

Whey Protein

Whey protein is protein in his purest form and is a good supplement to your daily protein intake. This type of protein isn't complicated and shouldn't be too expensive. A simple protein found at GNC or other health food chains should be sufficient.

Vitamin D

Vitamin D is an extremely important supplement that we need for a variety of different reasons. It is also very important for your metabolism, and it can help in different areas such as:

- Cancer prevention
- Fertility
- Insulin resistance
- Diabetes
- Cardiovascular disease
- Etc.

The most common way to get vitamin D into your system is through the sun. Yes, sunbathing or sun tanning can be a productive task after all. But, I know that laying out is sometimes impractical, especially for people who work and people who live in places like Seattle where it rains most of the year.

If you can sunbathe 15 to 30 minutes per day, I would try to do that. That is my preferred method if I can fit it in. If you can't fit that in, you can buy vitamin D supplements which will do just fine. You can find vitamin D at almost any supplement store, as well as Walmart, Target, etc.

Vitamin C

This is another vitamin that I take daily, and you should probably do so too. It has the effect of aiding in weight loss and helps your immune system as well. Overall, it's a good vitamin supplement to take when not eating as much fruit. You can find vitamin C at pretty much any drugstore, grocery store, or health food store.

Emergen-C packets are also great. Quick, easy, and delicious. You can find these almost anywhere.

Omega-3 Fats

We have already established that Omega-3 fats are extremely beneficial for your body, and how it is important to get the correct amount. But getting enough Omega-3 fats might be difficult with just raw foods. There are usually two varieties of fish oils – pharmaceutical grade or normal. If you can afford pharmaceutical grade, go with that; however, if you're tight on money, or on a budget, get a medium-priced fish oil.

Paleo Diet Eating Plan

You now have the basis for the Paleo diet lifestyle, and now it's time to implement it into your own life. I've put together a quick plan for you to stick to. It's not very complicated and I've kept it simple on purpose so it doesn't overwhelm you. Try your best to stick to this plan for 30 days and see how you feel (do I sound like a broken record yet?). I think you get the idea. JUST GO FOR IT!

Your Paleo meal plan for the next 30 days is actually quite simple. You are going to mix and match from each food group every single day for four meals per day (or whenever you are hungry).

Like I said so many times throughout this book, don't over complicate this. Just mix-and-match the right types of foods in each category: proteins, carbohydrates, and fats. You'll be choosing different foods within the Paleo guidelines, and within these categories, you can mix-and-match all day long.

Breakfast - Eggs are always a good starter to your day (unless you fall into the autoimmune category). Check the recipe section at the end of this section for other breakfast ideas including pancakes and omelets.

Examples:

Omelets with veggies and meat (bacon, turkey bacon, ham etc)
Egg scramble with meat and veggies (spinach, tomatoes, onions, bell peppers, etc.)
3 eggs and a fresh juice (Juicing recipes found at **FCRW.org/juicing**)

Lunch and Dinner are easy as well - use the shopping list from earlier in the book and use these items to make your lunch and dinner meals. I've also included several recipes at the end of this section, which will provide you with great tasty meal ideas for you and your family.

Choose a protein:
• chicken
• grass-fed steak
• shrimp
• pork chop
• beef patty
• tilapia (or any other fish)
• Etc.

Choose a Carb (i.e. veggie and/or fruit):
• Broccoli
• Asparagus

- Bell peppers
- Mushrooms
- Spinach
- Kale
- Etc.

Choose a Fat:
- Avocado
- Almonds
- Macadamia nuts
- Etc.

Examples:
- Chicken fajitas*
- Chicken curry*
- Pork curry*
- Pork roast*

Note* - check next section for full recipes.

Typical Paleo Day Example

Ok... here is an example day for those of you who want an example. I want to stress that this is just an example. Like I said before, you should never feel hungry on the paleo diet. If you are hungry, EAT FOOD! Obviously stick to the right foods, but make sure you are "fueled" up at all times. If you aren't hungry, you don't have to eat. Simple, right?

Breakfast
Olive oil in a pan
3-5 eggs scrambled
2-4 strips turkey bacon
1/2 - 1 Avocado

Snack 1
Apple with 10 almonds (eating them together
almost tastes like a candied apple - it's really good)

Lunch
Chicken breast (baked in the oven or reheated)
1 cup broccoli
Handful of kale or spinach
1/2 avocado
6-10 cashews

Snack 2
2-4 celery sticks with cashew butter

Dinner
1-2 Salmon filets
1 cup Broccoli or cauliflower or asparagus
1 cup kale for a side salad drizzled with olive oil
and lemon
1/2 avocado or 5-7 walnuts

Dessert
Healthy smoothie or 90% dark chocolate (only eat
dessert if you are craving sugar)

That's it! Eating this way keeps you feeling satisfied longer because of the healthy fat and protein intake, which will give you more energy and allow you to focus on more important things, like spending time with your family or picking up a new hobby.

Paleo Recipes

Eating Paleo doesn't necessarily have to be boring. Here are 21 of my favorite Paleo recipes. They're not in any particular order, but they are all amazing! I also have two Paleo cookbooks out that have an additional 30+ recipes! My Paleo Dinner recipe book is extremely cheap at the moment.

Go to ---> **FCRW.org/dinner**

Paleo Breakfast Recipes

Western Style Omelet

Omelets are one of the best and easiest breakfast items you can make. They taste delicious and aren't that hard to make. This is a Western-style omelet with all the ingredients to make a delicious start to your day.

Serves 2

Ingredients:

- 6 eggs
- Olive oil
- 1/2 cup chopped onion
- 1/2 cup chopped bell peppers
- 1/2 cup chopped tomato
- 1 cup spinach
- 4 ounces diced ham
- Sea salt and black pepper to taste

Preparation:

1. Crack all the eggs and put into a bowl, beat well.

2. Pour half the eggs into a non-stick skillet covered with a table spoon of olive oil.
3. Cook over medium heat.
4. When eggs have begun to set, add half of the chopped veggies and ham to one side of the eggs.
5. Using a spatula (silicon preferably), fold into half over the ham and veggies. Cook for 1 to 2 minutes longer, season with salt and pepper and serve.

Almond Banana Pancakes

Breakfast items are pretty straightforward, but every now and then it's good to mix it up with a little something special. This is where almond banana pancakes come into play.

Serves 2

Ingredients:

- 4 ripe bananas, mashed
- 2 eggs
- 4 tablespoons almond butter
- Butter or coconut oil for cooking

Preparation:

1. Combine the mashed bananas in a bowl with the eggs and mix well. Add the almond butter and combine well.
2. Put a pan over medium heat and melt in some butter or coconut oil. When hot, poor a ladle full of the banana and almond batter mixture and cook until brown on each side.

Sausage Stir-Fry For Breakfast

Here is another breakfast item for you to try. If you like sausage, then this might be the dish for you. Very tasty, and easy to make.

Serves 2-3

Ingredients:

- 1 to 2 teaspoons olive oil
- 1/2 cup diced onions
- 1/4 pound sausages, sliced
- 4 cups of spinach or other greens

Preparation:

1. Add olive oil to a skillet.
2. Heat over medium heat.
3. Add diced onions, sauté until soft. Add the sausage, cook until browned, tossing occasionally.
4. Add the greens, reduce the heat to medium low and cover.
5. Stir greens until they become soft.

Quick Paleo Pancakes

Here is another version of Paleo pancakes you can make in the morning. This is good if you have kids or if you are just looking for something different.

Serves 2-3

Ingredients:

- 2 eggs
- 1/2 cup unsweetened applesauce
- 1/2 cup nut butter (not peanut butter - cashew, almond, macadamia are great)
- 1/4 teaspoon cinnamon
- 1/4 teaspoon vanilla extract
- Coconut oil

Preparation:

1. Mix all the ingredients except the coconut oil into a bowl.
2. Stir well, until you have a semi-thick batter.
3. Next, use a little bit of coconut oil to grease a nonstick skillet.
4. Spread some of the batter into the skillet to form a pancake, and cook over low to medium heat.

5. Flip after 1-2 minutes, being careful not to burn them.

Paleo Lunch Recipes

Chicken Fajitas

Chicken fajitas are one of the easiest and most delicious meals I make. I really love how they are easy to prepare and how delicious they are with the little effort you have to put into making them. I typically make fajitas at least two or three times a week.

Serves 5

Ingredients:

- 3 pounds chicken breast, cut into thin strips
- 3 Bell peppers
- 3 onions, sliced
- 1 tablespoon each: garlic salt, chili powder, cumin, coriander
- Six chopped garlic cloves
- Juice of five lemons
- 4 tablespoons cooking fat
- Lettuce wedges to replace tortillas.

Preparation:

1. Combine the chicken, bell peppers, onions, spices, garlic and lemon juice in a bowl and mix well.
2. When ready to cook, heat a large skillet over medium heat and cook the whole preparation with the cooking fat until chicken is cooked.
3. Put fajitas in a large bowl and put toppings on the table for people to prepare on their own.

Shrimp and Salmon Chowder

I love a little clam chowder every now and then, but this version makes it extra tasty and nutritious (and healthy to boot). If you are a seafood lover, this is the dish for you!

Serves 4

Ingredients:

- 15 large raw shrimps
- 3 slices of bacon
- 1 onion, finely chopped
- 1 tablespoon fresh dill, chopped
- 1 Bay leaf
- 2 celery stalks, finely chopped
- 2 cups chopped cauliflower
- 1 1/2 cups chicken stock
- 1 wild salmon fillet, cut into bite-size pieces
- 1 can coconut milk
- Sea salt and fresh ground pepper to taste

Preparation:

1. Over medium heat and a large sauce pan, cook the bacon until it starts to release it's fat. Add the onion, dill, bay leaf and season with salt and pepper to taste. Cook until the bacon is crispy.

2. Add the chicken stock, celery, cauliflower, bring to a simmer for about seven minutes or until vegetables are soft.

3. Add the coconut milk, raw shrimp and salmon pieces, and combine and simmer for another 8 to 10 minutes or until fish and shrimp are well cooked.

Canned Salmon Salad

This is an extremely easy meal to prepare. If you are busy or on the go, something fast and delicious like this recipe will do just the trick. Minimal ingredients, and no real cooking required makes this dish a go-to if you just don't feel like cooking :-)

Serves 2

Ingredients:

- 2 cans wild salmon
- 2 cucumbers, diced
- 1 onion, chopped
- 1 large tomato, diced
- 1 avocado, diced
- 5 - 6 tablespoons extra virgin olive oil
- Juice of two lemons
- Lettuce leaves

Preparation:

1. Drain the liquid from the canned salmon, place them in a bowl and mash well with a fork.
2. Add the lemon juice and olive oil and mix well into the salmon.
3. Add the cucumbers, onion, tomato, and avocado and mix again.
4. Chop salad and serve cold.

Stir-Fry Beef Salad

This is a really easy way to make a quick salad that is tasty and good for on-the-go meals.

Serves 2

Ingredients:

- 2 teaspoons olive oil
- 3/4 cup diced onion
- 1 pound beef tips steak, sliced into thin strips
- 1 tablespoon wheat free soy sauce
- 1 - 2 cups sliced bell peppers
- 1 bag of mixed greens
- Balsamic vinegar

Preparation:

1. Add olive oil to a skillet.
2. Heat over medium. Add sliced onions, sauté until soft.
3. Add the beef and soy sauce, tossing often.
4. Add the bell peppers when the beef is browned..
5. Add the mix greens to your plate and top with stir-fry meat. Add balsamic vinegar and olive oil to taste.

Chicken Curry

Sticking with our Thai theme for the time being, this chicken curry dish is extremely easy to make and really tasty. As with all the other dishes, this one is just as simple and tastes just as good.

Serves 2-4

Ingredients:

- 1/2 cup chopped onion
- 1 tablespoon olive oil
- 1 diced chicken breast or thigh
- 1/4 cup curry sauce
- 1/4 cup cashews
- 2 cups chopped spinach

Preparation:

1. Sauté onions in the olive oil until soft.
2. Add chicken, heat until cooked through.
3. Add the curry sauce and cashews, continue heating for 3 to 4 minutes.
4. Remove from heat, stir in the spinach and serve.

Easy Shrimp

This is a great dish for easy shrimp on the go when you don't have a lot of time to prepare a large meal. Very tasty as well!

Serves 3-4

Ingredients:

- 1 pound wild caught Argentinian red shrimp or other shrimp of your choice.
- 1 bag frozen roasted red bell peppers and onions.
- 4 big handfuls of baby spinach.
- 2 tablespoons coconut oil.
- 2 tablespoons coconut milk.
- 1/2 tablespoon curry powder.
- Sea salt and black pepper to taste.

Preparation:

1. In a large skillet, heat the coconut oil over medium heat.
2. And onions and bell peppers and cook until defrosted and sizzling if using the frozen variety.
3. Add the shrimp and the spinach and cook for 3 to 4 minutes.
4. Add the coconut milk and spices, mix well and serve.

Broccoli and Spicy Italian Sausage

This is a great recipe using a variety of broccoli and cauliflower called broccoflower. It serves as a rice substitute and it is very delicious.

Serves 2-4

Ingredients:

- 1 pound hot Italian sausage
- 1 broccoflower Florette
- 1 cup diced red bell pepper
- 1/2 cup chopped fresh parsley

Preparation:

1. Begin heating a large pot or Dutch oven over medium heat.
2. Remove the casing from the spicy Italian sausage.
3. Brown the sausage in the pan using a fork or spatula to break up into pieces.
4. Take your broccoflower florets and steam them until you get a desired consistency.
5. Placed the broccoflower in a food processor and pulse until approximately the size of rice.
6. Once the sausage is completely browned, add the "riced" broccoflower to the pan and stir well, cooking for about 5 to 10 minutes.

Cashew Thai Chicken Scramble

This dish is one of my favorites because it is easy to create and tastes absolutely delicious. I usually pre-cook my chicken in advance but you don't have to (It just makes it easier).

Ingredients:

- 1/4 cup liquid amino acids from Bragg's
- 2 tablespoons cashew butter
- 4 Boneless skinless chicken breasts
- 1 inch piece of ginger
- 3 tablespoons minced garlic
- 3 tablespoons red chili paste

Preparation:

1. Mix amino acids, minced garlic, and chili paste in a bowl.
2. Cut boneless chicken breasts into 1 inch cubes.
3. Drop chicken cubes into marinade sauce and mix together well or until coated (optional - marinate for 3 hours).
4. Add chicken pieces to large skillet and cook until browned on all sides.
5. Once chicken is browned, add in marinade sauce and cook until chicken is cooked through (about 7-10 minutes).
6. Add cashew butter to mixture and stir together, let simmer for 3-4 minutes.

7. Serve with steamed vegetables.

Paleo Dinner Recipes

Citrus Pork Rib Roast

This is a very delicious roast with a ton of flavor. Best served with vegetables.

Serves 5

Ingredients:

- One pork rib roast (4 pounds)
- Three garlic cloves
- Two lemons
- Two oranges
- 10 Bay leaves
- For rosemary sprigs
- 1 tablespoon fennel seeds (chopped)
- Half tablespoon juniper berries, crushed
- 2 tablespoon extra virgin olive oil
- Cooking fat

Preparation:

1. Make small incisions on the fatty side of the pork roast and insert a garlic clove in each of them.

2. Combine the olive oil, cooking fat, and the juice and zest of lemons and oranges in a baking dish together with the bay leaves, rosemary, fennel seeds and juniper berries.
3. Season with sea salt and pepper and place the roast in the marinade overnight.
4. Makes sure the roast is at room temperature before cooking the next day.
5. Preheat the oven to three 350°F
6. Brown the roast in a skillet on medium heat.
7. Place the roast in a clean baking dish and roast for about 1 1/2 hours or until a thermometer indicates 145°F in the thickest part.
8. Let roast sit for 15 minutes and serve.

Crockpot Beef and Sweet Potato Stew

On any diet or eating plan, the crockpot is actually one of your best friends if you can use it properly. I like anything that will allow me to multitask, so naturally, I like making meals in crockpots. This recipe incorporates two of my favorite food items, beef and sweet potatoes :-)

Ingredients:

- 1 pound beef chuck cut into 1 inch cubes
- 3 cups sweet potatoes, peeled and cut into 1 inch cubes
- 2 garlic cloves, minced
- 1 bay leaf
- 1 cinnamon stick
- 1 large onion, cut into chunks
- 1 can (28 ounces) tomatoes
- Chopped parsley for garnishing
- 2 tablespoons cooking fat
- Sea salt and freshly ground black pepper to taste

Preparation:

1. Heat a skillet over a medium heat, season the beef cubes to taste with salt and pepper and brown them on all sides with some cooking fat in a hot skillet.
2. Place the browned beef, sweet potatoes, garlic, cinnamon stick, onion, tomato, and garlic in the

crockpot and cook on low for eight hours or until beef is tender.

3. Remove cinnamon sticks and bay leaves when done.

Chicken Marsala

This dish is a great one to make when you're craving any type of European dish (i.e. French or Italian food). Typically, this dish is prepared with a marsala wine, however, any red wine or chicken stock will do.

Serves 4

Ingredients:

- 5 boneless chicken breasts
- 5 slices of bacon cut into 1 inch pieces
- 1/2 pound button mushrooms
- 1 garlic clove, minced
- 1 teaspoon tomato paste
- 1/2 cup marsala or other red wine
- 1 1/2 tablespoon lemon juice
- 4 tablespoons butter or Ghee, divided into four pieces
- 2 tablespoons fresh parsley
- 2 tablespoons cooking fat
- Sea salt or black pepper to taste

Preparation:

1. Heat some cooking fat in a large skillet over medium heat, season the chicken breast with salt and pepper and cook for about three

minutes on each side, until golden brown and cooked through.

2. Over a medium low heat, cook bacon for about four minutes or until crisp. Set the bacon aside for later.
3. Add the mushrooms to the skillet and cook for eight minutes on medium heat, until the liquid extracted from the mushrooms has evaporated entirely and the mushrooms are slightly browned.
4. Add the cooked bacon, garlic and tomato paste and cook for about one minute.
5. Add the Marsala or red wine, bring to a boil and cook until liquid is reduced to about 1 1/4 cups, or about five minutes.
6. Take the skillet off of the heat, add in the lemon juice and whisk in the butter or Ghee, one piece at a time.
7. Add the parsley and season to taste with salt and pepper.
8. Pour the marsala sauce over the cooked chicken and serve.

Paleo Spaghetti

I don't know about you, but I love Italian food.
The only bad thing, is that pasta and most Italian
dishes are not on the Paleo diet. But, have no fear!
- this is a recipe that is healthy and fits in with your
new Paleo lifestyle. Enjoy!

Serves 4

Ingredients:

- 1 pound ground beef or ground turkey
- 1 tablespoon olive oil
- 1 (12 oz) package of kelp noodles
- 1-2 cups marinara sauce
- 1-2 cloves of crushed garlic

Preparation:

1. Brown the meat in the olive oil using a large
   skillet.
2. When the meat is browned, add the kelp
   noodles and the marinara sauce.
3. Stir and bring to a simmer.
4. Add the crushed garlic just before serving.

Pork Curry

Thai food is one of my favorite foods in the world. This dish is extremely tasty and can be made fairly easily without having to go out and spend money at a Thai restaurant.

Serves 2-4

Ingredients:

- 1 pound ground pork
- 1 tablespoon olive oil
- 1-2 tablespoons curry powder
- 1 bag baby spinach
- 1/2 can coconut milk (7 ounces)
- 2-3 garlic cloves

Preparation:

1. In a large pot brown the pork in the olive oil.
2. Add the curry powder as the pork browns and mix well.
3. Break up any larger lumps of pork.
4. Once the pork is browned, add all the spinach and the coconut milk.
5. Heat until the spinach has cooked down.
6. Add the garlic at the end, either minced or using a garlic press to crush it.
7. Mix well, remove from heat and serve.

Paleo Chicken Alfredo

Once again, we are here with an Italian dish. Chicken Alfredo is one of the most tasty dishes in Italian cuisine (in my opinion). This dish takes it to another level and is really healthy.

Serves 2-4

Ingredients:

- 2 teaspoons olive oil
- 4 cloves of garlic, chopped
- 1 lb. chicken breast
- 1 (12 ounce) package of kelp noodles
- 2 teaspoons tarragon
- 1 cup cashews
- 1/2 teaspoon onion powder
- 1/4 teaspoon garlic powder
- 1/4 teaspoon mustard powder
- 1/4 teaspoon sea salt
- 1/4 teaspoon pepper
- 1/4 teaspoon paprika

Preparation:

1. Add the olive oil into a large skillet.
2. Sauté the garlic over medium heat for 3 to 4 minutes.

3. Chop the chicken into 1 inch cubes, and add to the skillet and cook until browned on both sides.
4. Rinse and chop the kelp noodles. Add them to the skillet along with the tarragon, cover and cook on low for 30 minutes.
5. Pour the liquid from the skillet carefully into a small container for use in the sauce.
6. Add the cashews, onion powder, garlic powder, mustard powder, salt, pepper, and paprika to a blender.
7. Cover and blend into a powder.
8. Add the reserved pan juices after (slowly), blending into a thick sauce.
9. Use a spatula to scrape up the sides of the blender.
10. Add the juices until the mixture reaches your desired consistency.
11. Add the sauce to skillet the mix well. Cover and continue to cook for 10 minutes longer to kelp noodles have become tender.

Paleo Dessert Recipes

Macadamia and Avocado Smoothie

Serves 1

Ingredients:

- 1/2 cup coconut milk
- 1/2 avocado
- 1/2 cup strawberries
- 5 macadamia nuts or 1 tablespoon macadamia butter
- 1/2 cup water
- 1-2 tablespoons raw honey or other natural sweetener
- 2 ice cubes

Preparation:

1. Put all ingredients into a blender. Blend until smooth. Serve immediately.

Chocolate Paleo Snack Cake Recipe

Serves 2-4

Ingredients:

- 10 medjool dates, pitted
- 1 cup unsweetened applesauce or one ripe banana
- 3 eggs
- 1/2 cup coconut oil
- 2 teaspoons vanilla extract
- 1/2 cup coconut flour
- 1/2 cup unsweetened cocoa powder
- 1 teaspoon baking soda
- 1/2 teaspoon fine sea salt
- 1/2 cup strong grade coffee

Preparation:

1. Place the dates in a food processor and pulse until puréed.
2. Add applesauce and continue to pulse until puréed and combine with the dates.
3. Add fruit purée to the bowl of a stand mixer, add the eggs, vanilla, coconut oil and coffee and mix on low/medium speed until well combined.
4. Combine the dry ingredients in a separate bowl.

5. Slowly add the dry ingredients into the wet ingredients and mix on low speed, scraping the sides, until you have a smooth mixture.
6. Bake at 350°F for 30 to 35 minutes or until a toothpick stuck in the middle comes out clean.

Paleo Mocha Chocolate Chip Cookies

Ingredients:

- 2 1/3 cups almond flour
- 1/2 cup cocoa powder
- 1/2 teaspoon sea salt
- 1/2 teaspoon baking soda
- 1 packet espresso powder
- 1 tablespoon vanilla extract
- 1/2 cup coconut oil or butter melted
- 1/2 cup coconut nectar or sweetener of choice
- 3/4 cup dark chocolate chips

Preparation:

1. Preheat oven to 350°F.
2. Combine dry ingredients in a large bowl.
3. Combine what ingredients in a small bowl.
4. Mix wet ingredients into dry ingredients.
5. Use a small cookie dough scoop or form into 1/2 inch balls and place on a parchment paper lined cookie sheet.
6. Press down onto pan to form round discs or cookie shapes.
7. Bake for 10 minutes.
8. Remove and cool.

Conclusion

Thank you very much for reading this Paleo Diet book. I hope you now understand how the Paleo diet can change your lifestyle and give you a more abundant life full of energy. My hope is that you take the next 30 days and put all of this Paleo diet information into practice, and see how you feel at the end of those 30 days. I am confident that you'll feel amazing at the end of this trial period! Here's to your health!

Would You Do Me A Quick Favor?

If you liked this book and found it helpful, (liked a recipe, learned something new, etc), I would really appreciate it if you left a review on Amazon for me. Trust me...your support on Amazon means the world to me! It really helps me out, and I read every single review.

If you didn't like something about the book I would love for you to PLEASE email me before leaving a review: ryantaylorhealth@gmail.com. This way I can make changes to the book and make it better for future readers!

Just log in and click the button that says "create your own review" at the top of the page. Takes 1 minute :)

FREE Paleo Breakfast Recipe Book!

For a limited time I am giving away my Best Selling Paleo Breakfast Recipe Book for FREE! Yes, that's right... head to **FreeBookGift.com** now!

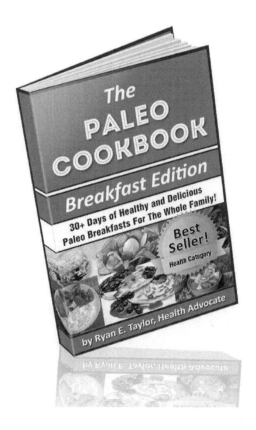

More Best Sellers That Compliment The Paleo Diet:

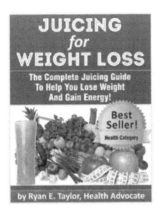

GO Here--> **FCRW.org/juicing**

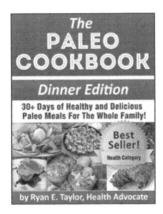

GO Here--> **FCRW.org/dinner**

Made in the USA
San Bernardino, CA
20 February 2014